Approach and Talk to Women Easily: The How to Talk to Girls Masterclass

By Craig Beck

www.CraigBeck.com

Forward

Picture this. The most stunning woman you have ever seen walks past you in Starbucks. You feel the spark, the pull, that quiet voice screaming go and talk to her. But your feet stay glued to the floor. She leaves. You go home alone. Again.

Every single day, gorgeous, available, intelligent women cross your path. In the supermarket queue. On the train platform. At the gym. Walking the dog. And every single day, ordinary guys watch those opportunities evaporate because they were too scared to say hello.

This book ends that.

Forget cheesy pickup lines. Forget memorised routines. Forget peacocking and silly games that only work at 2am when everyone is drunk and the lights are low. Out here in the real world, in daylight, sober, you must approach as the confident, warm, intelligent man you already are underneath the fear.

This is a full daytime cold approach masterclass from a leading expert in persuasion and human behaviour. You will learn how to walk up to any woman, anywhere, and create instant attraction. Not through tricks. Through psychology.

Inside you will discover:

How to crush approach anxiety in under sixty seconds.
The exact words to open with, and how to deliver them.
FBI-grade body language tactics that broadcast high-value confidence before you even open your mouth.
How to flip rejection into rocket fuel.

The art of becoming the most memorable moment of her entire day.
Proven techniques to take the conversation from hello to her number, the date, and beyond.

The men who get the women, the careers, the life they want are not better looking, richer, or smarter than you. They simply learned one skill. The skill to approach.

Today is the day you learn it too.

Buy now. Read it tonight. Approach her tomorrow.

www.CraigBeck.com

The Rules of Engagement

You may think that attractive women are constantly approached by guys. However, the reality often contradicts this common assumption. Most men simply lack the confidence to put themselves out there. Even in traditional dating settings like bars and clubs, many men require a few drinks to gather the courage to approach a girl.

This book doesn't focus on those environments; instead, it explores daytime opportunities to meet beautiful girls that arise every day. These situations are real and often present genuine challenges for men to overcome their fears. Unlike a nightclub, where guys are expected to make advances, this is different. You're truly stepping out of your comfort zone and making a bold statement in a non-traditional environment.

In a nightclub, virtually every woman expects to be hit on. In fact, many would be offended if they weren't approached. Put yourself in her shoes for a moment. Imagine spending hours getting ready, meticulously planning every detail from your outfit's color combination to your hairstyle, accessories, jewelry, and makeup. Then, after all that effort, not a single guy finds you attractive enough to approach. As men, we may struggle to grasp this concept because it's usually different for us. We can get by with a shower, a shave, a nice shirt, and our favorite pants. We're more likely to experience this type of rejection when we're already in a relationship. I remember a few years ago, when my girlfriend at the time arranged for us to visit an art gallery with her work colleagues. The dress code was smart casual, but I decided to impress her. I went to the hairdresser, got a professional shave at a local Turkish barber, picked out my favorite suit, pressed it, and paired it with a stylish pair of Italian leather shoes. I

completed the look with my most elegant Breitling watch and examined myself in the mirror.
I'll admit that when I'm in a relationship, I tend to lean toward a constant jeans-and-t-shirt look. So, I was feeling quite proud of how I had dressed up for my girl, and I had high expectations for her reaction. However, when I knocked on her front door and took a step back, eagerly awaiting the flood of praise and admiration, I have to confess that I was more than crushed when she didn't even notice. She glanced at me and said, "Oh, good, you're here. Let's get going so we can find a parking space." This is the kind of rejection women face every day.

Approaching women when they're in a social mindset will be covered in a different book. Right here and now, we're focusing on approaching girls when they least expect it or aren't consciously prepared for advances. In my personal opinion, this puts you in a much stronger position than when you're competing with other guys (like in a nightclub) and when her defenses are up. What I'm saying is that a woman waiting to be served at the bar in a club expects to be hit on, whereas a girl choosing pasta sauce in the supermarket doesn't—and it's this status quo that we can leverage to our advantage.

To approach women in daylight, non-social environments, there are seven important elements to consider:

- Preparation
- Timing
- Observation
- Delivery
- Detachment
- Closing
- Repetition

I will delve into each step in detail, but it's crucial to understand that each point is important. If you want to be successful, you can't afford to be weak in any of these areas.

Preparation

There is no doubt about it, approaching a hot woman is the most difficult aspect of the whole process but the approach on its own is not going to get you her number. If you walk up to a woman and just stare at her the chances are she will be reaching for her cell phone for an entirely different purpose. You need to be prepared to have a conversation with her. What I do not mean is that you have a rehearsed pick up line ready to go. Sure it's handy to have a few 'openers' that you can fall back on but in the most part an observation or question is more likely to portray you as a genuine guy rather than the stereotypical cheesy lounge lizard who uses pick up routines.

We will talk about this in more detail when we get to point three but I will state it here as well because it is so important. Your observation should never be a physical or sexual one. Do not ever tell the girl with amazing long legs that she has amazing long legs. It is blindingly predictable, paints you in a very bad light and automatically raises her shields to DEFCON 5.

Notice something unique about her or what she is doing. When I advise women on how to talk to hot guys I give an example of a practically bulletproof environment where any woman can approach a guy and get away with it. Guys in clothes shops always appreciate the advice of girls. I tell ladies to notice what the guy is looking at and genuinely tell him how he would look in that particular item of clothing. I suggest they can say things like 'You should definitely buy that, the color is perfect for your skin tone'. Guys are pretty slow at realizing that they are being hit on and so there is always an easy escape from the situation if the woman decides not to proceed any further (perhaps he is not quite as hot close up). They can always throw in the old 'my boyfriend has the same top and he has a similar build to you'. Although due to the law of scarcity that we talked about in the first book this often can have the opposite effect as intended.

Summary: Be prepared to talk, have something to say, have an opinion and have questions. You may very well have to lead the conversation but talking at the woman is not the objective. Your goal is to engage her in conversation, so that she enjoys talking to you and sharing her opinions with the nice friendly guy she just met.

Timing

Approach anxiety is real and it is the thing most likely to prevent you from getting a girl's number. Hey, if you don't approach at all, your chances of success are a guaranteed zero. Even if you approach the most beautiful woman on planet earth who is out shopping with her millionaire boyfriend, you have a better chance of scoring than the girl you didn't approach at all.

When you spot a beautiful woman, overthinking is your biggest enemy; don't give yourself time to think about what you're about to do. Your brain is hard-wired to protect you from harm, and I don't just mean physical injury. Emotional pain is something you discovered to be quite hurtful very early on in life, and you have developed subconscious mechanisms to protect yourself from experiencing it again. If you wait too long after seeing the woman, I guarantee you will come up with an endless stream of reasons why you should not approach her.

A few examples of the excuses your brain comes up with to try and protect you:

She looks busy; I would be inconveniencing her.
She is too attractive to be interested in me.
She is probably in a relationship.
I bet she gets hit on all the time.
What if I stumble and sound stupid?
What if she just stares at me like I'm some freak?
What if she rejects me?
What if she just laughs at me?
All these thoughts are 100% pure excuses designed to keep you away from potentially uncomfortable situations. Your brain has learned that touching a hot stove will burn you, and as a result, alarm bells start ringing when you approach it to keep you safe. The same thing happens

when you procrastinate over approaching a hot woman. Your subconscious programming is in a battle with your conscious desire. The main difference is that the hot stove will always hurt you if you touch it. Approaching girls you're attracted to may have the potential to be painful, but the more you do it, the less likely that outcome becomes. On the other hand, no matter how many times you touch the hot stove, the outcome won't improve.

So let's break down some of those "reasons" not to approach the girl and see what they really mean.

She looks busy; I would be inconveniencing her!
Yes, she may well be busy, but put yourself in her shoes. Can you imagine if you were running late for work and a hot girl stopped you to tell you how great you looked? Would you be annoyed at her? Unlikely. Your objective in approaching a woman is not just to get her number or manipulate her into bed. It is always about having a positive interaction with another human being. Your goal should be to make her day suddenly and significantly better. If you approach her, make her smile, and then she has to leave because she's in a rush, I would argue that this is a successful and positive event for both of you.

She is too attractive to be interested in me!
Firstly, you need to be aware of the different ways that men and women experience attraction. Men are primarily motivated by visual stimuli; we see a girl with amazing legs and we want her. While women are also attracted to what they see, it is not their primary focus. Females are generally much more attuned to how they feel about someone, they are motivated by emotions. So unless she is aware of your personality, confidence, and character, you have no idea if she is "too attractive" for you or not.

Most importantly, you need to understand that 99.9% of guys will NEVER have the courage to approach her for this very reason/excuse. She doesn't get hit on nearly as much as you think, and most guys are so bad at approaching girls that half the time the woman in question isn't even aware of what is going on.

Last year in Cyprus (where I currently live), I was in a hotel reception and the girl working behind the desk was the most beautiful woman I had ever seen in my life. I started talking to her and quickly discovered that she was married to a soldier who was based at the British army garrison in Dhekelia. I told her what I did and all about the book I was writing, and I asked her roughly how many times a week she gets hit on. She looked stunned and said, "Oh God, I don't know. I don't think it's as often as that." I suspect that she actually gets hit on nearly every day, but the approaches are so bad that she doesn't even acknowledge them.

What you must understand is that most men who see a beautiful woman wouldn't dream of approaching her for fear of rejection. Maybe 1% will attempt a half-hearted approach, but they do it so poorly that the girl won't have the slightest idea what they're doing. The remaining rare guys who do have "game" and know they are operating in a very small but lucrative pond. This is where I want you to join the party, in the top 1% of all men.

Additionally, with this excuse to avoid approaching, you are assuming that the woman knows she is beautiful. There are very few people, male or female, who can look in the mirror and be totally happy with what they see. In my experience, people who fall into this tiny minority are best avoided anyway. The chances are good that the girl of your desires doesn't see herself with quite the halo that you do in that moment.

She is probably in a relationship!
Or she probably isn't. The truth is that you won't know for sure until you get to know her. Even if she is in a relationship, it doesn't have to be the end of the game. Personally, I've never been comfortable trying to tempt a girl into cheating. Whether you continue to pursue a sexual conquest after learning this information is entirely your choice, and I certainly don't judge you for it. Hey, we're all adults here, and it really does take two to tango. Some women are looking for that kind of no-strings excitement, and if it works for you too, then go for it.

But the most important point I want to make in response to this excuse not to approach is that if you think her availability has the power to ruin your interaction with her, then you're missing the point of "game," in my humble opinion. Not every approach has to lead to getting a phone number, not every phone number will lead to a date, and not every date will end in sex. The primary objective of approaching a beautiful woman is because it's fun and you get to meet someone who is hopefully as amazing on the inside as she is on the outside.

If you approach a married woman, flatter her, make her feel special, and have a fun conversation with her before you both go your separate ways, who loses anything? If you get it right, then you almost certainly made her day, and she will have an extra spring in her step as a result of what you did. You had a fun conversation with a beautiful woman and got to practice your approach.

Remember, no matter how many times you touch the hot stove, it will always hurt. Approach anxiety is different; it gets better every time you approach a girl, whether you get the desired result or not.

Finally, let me describe the worst-case scenario in this situation. It's a scenario I know well because it happened to me in London a few years ago. A stunningly attractive woman turned off Regent Street and walked into an upscale department store. I noticed her immediately, and the countdown started in my head. By the count of three, I had my hand on her elbow, stopping her with a smile. As soon as I started talking, I became aware of her husband, who had been a few feet in front of her. He had noticed me talking to his wife and had doubled back to make his presence felt. Our eyes met just as I was telling his wife that she had great style and had really caught my eye. I quickly turned my attention to him and said, "Is this your wife?" He grunted an emotionless "yes," and I smiled my biggest smile yet, saying, "Wow, you are a lucky guy."

I said it was nice to meet them both and walked back out onto Regent Street. What do you think happened next?

Did the guy start an argument with his wife?
Did he chase after me and punch me in the face?
Did he call the police?

Yes, that's right. He chased after me and punched my lights out. No, just kidding! Of course, he didn't attack me, but why not?

The simple answer is that I wasn't being disrespectful. I approached in a friendly and fun way. I didn't try to disrespect him, and I included him in the conversation (whether he liked it or not) as soon as he entered the scene. I wasn't rude or inappropriate; I simply told him that he was a lucky guy and that his wife was beautiful. I might have rubbed his alpha male ego the wrong way, but deep down inside, he was probably pretty proud of himself.

So even in the worst-case scenario, nothing particularly unpleasant happens. So stop using "she's probably in a relationship" as an excuse to avoid approaching!

What if I stumble or sound stupid?

What! Are you crazy? Hugh Grant has made a career out of it. Okay, seriously, nobody wants to come across as nervous or lacking confidence, but worrying about it actually creates the situation you're trying to avoid. The best way to consistently improve in this area is to do lots of approaches. Approach, approach, and approach until you can do it without thinking. I'm just like you; I had to learn this stuff. I wasn't born with "game"; I had mentors who taught me what to do, and some of them were badass drill sergeants of "game." Some days when I was learning, I would make over 50 approaches. When I first started, I would also get about 45 rejections a day. Nothing hurts quite like nearly 50 hot girls saying no or worse to you in a single day. The next day, you feel beaten up, and the last thing you want to do is make another approach. All you want to do is crawl under your duvet and hide. But something magical happens while you're asleep. Your subconscious absorbs vast amounts of data while you were busy being rejected, and what you'll almost always find is that the next day is better, often dramatically better. I have personally been rejected dozens of times on a Saturday, only to have a 100% success rate the very next day, going home with a dozen phone numbers. So many that I can't even remember which one was which.

I like what Ross Jeffries suggests as a way to overcome the excuse of "what if I say something stupid." He actually tells guys to deliberately go up to girls and say the dumbest thing they can think of. In one of his YouTube videos, he advises people to go up to the hottest woman they can find and ask, "Hey, what's your favorite flavor of a bowling ball?" The reason is simple: There's no point worrying about saying something stupid if you already know that's exactly what you intend to do.

Keep approaching, and whatever you do, don't stop. Occasionally, you're going to say something dumb, but it's not brain surgery, nobody dies, and you'll get another chance to try again within a few minutes.

What about rejection?

I'm going to group the final three excuses into one because they're all variations on the theme of rejection.

Everyone fears rejection; it's completely natural and understandable. But that doesn't mean that this mindset protects you or serves you in any way. Let's understand where this fear comes from and why it's so powerful in our lives today. The fear of rejection kicks in from the moment we're born, and rightfully so. Rejection at this point in our lives could result in death. We're born completely helpless, unable to perform even the most basic functions needed to sustain life. We can't even eat or drink without someone taking care of us. Later in life, when we leave the safety of our family home and venture out into the world of school and social interactions, we discover that being accepted feels good, but we also learn how painful social rejection can be. From birth to around the age of seven, the information we absorb is deeply wired into our subconscious mind and influences much of our personality and character. Any deep-seated phobias and fears that you can't explain were probably created and repressed during this time. Essentially, the brain is in its formative stage and doesn't have enough data to filter the incoming information. If you tell a 4-year-old that the earth is flat, they will most likely believe you. Why wouldn't they? They probably haven't encountered lies and deceit at this early point in their life, and they have no evidence to argue against what you're claiming.

During this early stage of our lives, we learn at an incredible pace. Most of what we learn serves us in a positive way, but a significant amount of the data can hinder us later on. One of these faulty programs is the belief that rejection is something to be feared or that we need the approval of others to be happy. This belief is deeply ingrained but entirely untrue.

In the context of dating, this manifests as approach anxiety and worrying about our advances being declined or, worse, laughed at. Gravity is real, and we can prove that by attempting to defy it. No matter how many times you jump in the air, you won't succeed in floating off into space. The fear of rejection is not based on truth, and we can prove this by repeatedly exposing ourselves to it. To overcome your fear of approaching women, you have to confront the very thing you're most afraid of, not just once but dozens, if not hundreds, of times. This is the only way to overcome this self-limiting mindset.

The reality of life is that significant growth and progress happen when you operate outside your comfort zone. True learning occurs when you're in uncomfortable and unfamiliar territory. In the context of seduction, it means pushing yourself into situations that genuinely challenge you. You can spend a lifetime cautiously approaching average-looking women, but you'll never reach your true potential. You have to approach the women you feel have zero chance with, the ones you consider 9/10. It may be painful, but it's the fastest and most effective way to develop the skills you desire.

Many years ago, when I was training in the field with another pickup artist, we visited a nightclub in London. As we entered the club, I was told that I couldn't choose who to approach that evening. I would be instructed on who to approach, and I was warned that if I refused at any point, the evening would be over, and I would be back in my hotel bed alone before the night even began. My first approach of the evening was a scenario so ridiculous it could give a grown man recurring nightmares. I stood on the edge of the dance floor with my mentor, surveying the possible approaches in the club. I pointed to a somewhat cute girl dancing alone and looking a little lost. My coach frowned and shook his head. I pointed to a group of girls who were clearly intoxicated and on their way to oblivion, and again he firmly shook his head. Then he raised his hand, pointed to the center of the dance floor, and said, "Her, she's yours."

I looked but couldn't figure out who he was pointing at, and then my heart sank. Surely he couldn't be suggesting what I had just considered. Unfortunately, I had correctly identified my target. A stunningly beautiful woman who was not only (in my opinion) way out of my league, but she was also already dancing and making out with another guy.

I turned to my coach and complained, "How the hell can I approach her? She's already with a guy. You're going to get me beaten up!" My mentor smiled and said, "That's not going to happen. Nobody has the balls to do what you're about to do. That guy is going to be shocked by how confident you are, and he's going to back off."

I stared at my target in disbelief at what I was about to do. I won't lie to you; in that moment, I was terrified. But I followed my mentor's instructions. Shockingly, exactly what he had predicted happened. The guy took a step back as I started talking to the girl, and within thirty seconds, he was nowhere to be seen. He had left the girl and me alone in the center of the dance floor.

Push through your self-imposed barriers, and you'll find that magical outcomes await you on the other side. Trust me on this—I've experienced both sides, and I can tell you from experience that being a member of the elite 1% is the life you want to live.

Observation

A lot of people claim that "Day Game" is more difficult and complicated than the traditional social environment of "Night Game," but I strongly disagree. It's not necessarily more difficult; it's just different and requires some special awareness. You have to put in a little more effort and be more genuine, but why is that a bad thing?

So, imagine you see an attractive woman walking through the mall. Ask yourself why it's absolutely necessary for you to approach her and start a conversation. If your answer is simply because she's attractive, then you're giving yourself a very poor chance of success. Approaching someone solely based on their physical appearance and telling them they're beautiful is like telling a swimmer they'll get wet in the water. It's obvious and doesn't say much about you. In fact, it conveys that you see yourself as inferior to her. Women are subconsciously programmed to seek value in men, and by making such an obvious statement about her appearance, you're positioning yourself as someone beneath her.

You might be tempted to use the opposite approach, commonly known as "negging." This technique involves giving backhanded compliments like, "Nice dress, it must be on sale because I've seen three girls today wearing the exact same dress," or "I love your nails, are they real?" I'm not a fan of negging, whether in night game or day game. This theory seems to stem from insecurity, suggesting that women need to be tricked or undermined to be attracted. Personally, I don't want to manipulate a woman into bed; I want her to be with me because she genuinely thinks I'm a cool guy and enjoys spending time with me.

Instead of trying to knock her confidence down to elevate yourself, avoid telling beautiful women that they're beautiful. Also, keep in mind that men are primarily visually stimulated, so the first thing you notice about her may not be the most important aspect in her mind. If you approach a girl with long legs and make them the focus of your opening approach, you'll likely be labeled as just another guy trying to pursue her for superficial reasons. Open your eyes and try to see her character and personality. Look for something unique about her that most guys would overlook because they're too busy checking out her physical attributes. Perhaps she has great style, a distinctive tattoo, a funny slogan on her t-shirt, or unique spectacles that suit her face. It doesn't matter what it is; make it personal and genuinely appreciate that aspect about her.

If you tell a girl that her bag is the coolest you've ever seen, make sure you genuinely mean it. If you're being dishonest, she might catch you in the lie or sense your insincerity. Either way, you're sabotaging the rapport before making any progress, and she'll likely put up her defenses and reject you.

Summary: Open your eyes and observe the girl and the world she lives in. Identify a unique characteristic you genuinely appreciate about her before approaching. It's not about fixating on her physical appearance; rather, it's about appreciating her as a whole person. Women are perceptive and sensory-aware, and they quickly pick up on your true state of mind.

Delivery

There's nothing more attractive to a woman than a confident man. Conversely, if you approach a hot woman and mumble something quietly, one or more of four things are likely to happen:

She will ask you to repeat what you said.
Her body language will change to a defensive posture because a stranger is acting in a secretive or covert manner around her.
She will feel uncomfortable in your presence.
She will feel sorry for you.
None of these outcomes are helpful. Remember, in daytime approaches, it's crucial to demonstrate confidence and your value as a real man. To achieve this, you need to approach her in a friendly yet assertive manner. If she's walking along the sidewalk, don't walk alongside her, as that gives her the power. Instead, step in front of her with a smile, pause her forward momentum, and speak loudly, clearly, and slowly. I'm not suggesting shouting in her face, but speak at a volume that conveys your comfort and confidence in what you're doing. You're doing something brave, something that 99% of guys wouldn't have the guts to do. Moreover, you don't care who sees you or what they think.

Let me share a quick story to illustrate this point. A few years ago, I approached a stunning woman in London, and a lady passing by interrupted me and said, "My God, you've got balls! Good for you, son." Her comment actually did me a favor because it further enhanced my image as a confident guy doing something out of the ordinary.

When you're nervous, there's a tendency to speak faster than usual. This happens because your subconscious senses that you're in a "dangerous" situation and tries to get you out of it as quickly as possible. Due to the rush of adrenaline and your focus on the mission, you may not even realize how fast you're talking until you stumble or see a confused expression on her face. Talking too quickly also tends to raise the pitch of your voice. To demonstrate confidence, you need to slow down your delivery, allowing you to express yourself confidently while lowering the pitch of your voice.

Here's a bonus secret for you: Back when I used to coach professional radio and TV presenters, I would emphasize the power of silence. Surprisingly, one of the most impactful demonstrations of confidence while speaking is when you say absolutely nothing. A deliberate pause within a sentence can be incredibly alluring. Imagine if I whispered in your ear that I know a dirty secret about you but paused for a few seconds before revealing it. The pause fuels intrigue, intensifying the emotions you're feeling.

Let's consider an example of approaching a hot woman in the street with two different delivery approaches. First, without a pause, and then adding the power of silence:

"Hey, I saw you crossing the street just now, and I noticed something about you. You have the coolest jeans I've ever seen. Where did you get them?"
"Hey, [PAUSE] I saw you crossing the street just now, and I noticed something about you [PAUSE]. You have the coolest jeans I've ever seen. Where did you get them?"
Do you see the power of the pause in the second approach? It creates a moment of anticipation and engages her imagination. In that momentary pause, she'll generate multiple possible responses in her mind. She won't be able to resist doing this; it's an automatic function of the conscious mind. By saying, "I noticed something about you," during the pause, you trigger her to come up with various thoughts, ranging from self-doubts like "Do I have a stain on my dress?" to protective assumptions like "He's going to comment on my long legs" to hopeful possibilities that you noticed something she put effort into, like a new hairstyle. The power of silence should not be

underestimated; it's incredibly magnetic when used effectively.

Finally, let's discuss body language for delivery. This aspect is often overlooked because many guys solely focus on what to say. You've probably heard the statistic that human communication consists of 55% body language, 31% tone of voice, and only 7% actual words. So, neglecting body language is a major mistake. If you approach a girl while feeling nervous but fail to consciously control your body language, it won't matter what you say or how you say it—your body will reveal the truth. Body language deserves an in-depth exploration, but here are a few things to watch out for:

Pay attention to your feet. They reveal where you want to be. If someone talks to me, and their legs or feet are pointed away from me, I instantly assume they'd rather not be engaged in conversation and want to be somewhere else.
If the woman you're talking to has her feet crossed in any way, it's a positive sign. It indicates that she's comfortable with you and doesn't feel the need to prepare for a quick escape. This is a good indicator of interest.
Scratching your nose or ears is a sign of discomfort. If you're not at ease during the conversation, she'll perceive it as a lack of confidence. People tend to touch their noses when they're lying because the brain activates certain erectile tissues in uncomfortable situations, and the nose is the most exposed area for this reaction. This sensation prompts us to reach and touch the concerned area, which becomes an obvious giveaway.
Watch out for comforting behaviors. When we're uneasy, we tend to exhibit baby-like actions such as stroking our hair, gripping the back of our neck, or fidgeting with items in our pockets. These subconscious indicators of unease don't convey confidence. Confident alpha males aren't

threatened by their surroundings, especially not by talking to attractive women. So, ditch these pacifying behaviors.
Summary:

Speak loudly with a calm and resonant voice.
Use pauses and inflections to demonstrate confidence.
Be a leader, not a follower. When approaching a walking woman, don't walk alongside her; make her stop and engage with you.
Utilize false time constraints to show that other people are waiting for you elsewhere.
Be nonchalant about her looks and playfully tease her.
Adopt a "take it or leave it" attitude. Don't be overly attached to any outcome and go with the flow, accepting acceptance and rejection with equal ease.

Detachment

One commonality we all share is the desire to feel happy and avoid pain. Yet, we often find ourselves in situations that set us up for pain. We attach our happiness to people, circumstances, and things, holding onto them tightly. We stress about the possibility of losing them when things don't go as expected. However, in approaching women, it's essential to release the fear of rejection because it is illogical.

We tend to attach our identity to our emotions, not just the positive ones but also negative ones like regret or disappointment. It can feel safe and even comforting to wallow in these negative emotions. By trying to hold onto what's familiar, we limit our ability to experience joy in the present. When we stop trying to grasp, own, and control the world around us, we give it the freedom to fulfill us without the power to destroy us. That's why letting go is crucial—it allows happiness to enter.

Letting go of attachment is not a one-time decision like ripping off a Band-Aid. It's an ongoing commitment, a day-to-day and moment-to-moment practice that involves changing how we experience and interact with the things we instinctively want to hold onto.

When it comes to rejection, it's important not to take it as a personal assault. Imagine making breakfast and reaching into the cutlery drawer to grab a spoon. You choose one spoon to use, but it doesn't mean you reject the other spoons. You don't feel guilty for leaving them in the drawer. Similarly, if a woman doesn't give you her number or outright rejects you, it's perfectly fine. It's her right to do so, and while it may bruise your ego and feel like a win/lose situation, it's actually a win/win scenario. Let me explain why.

Firstly, you don't know the exact reason why she rejected you. It's easy for your wounded ego to engage in self-pity, but there could be innocent reasons for her disinterest. Perhaps she just got fired from work, was in a rush to get somewhere, or had a bad day. We could speculate a hundred different possibilities, so beating yourself up and thinking you're not attractive, funny, or good enough is pointless.

It's crucial to detach yourself from the outcome and find value in rejection. Every time you approach a girl and fail to close the deal, consider it a valuable lesson. What you learn in that moment is worth more than hundreds of dollars. You'll learn far more from repeated approaches and experiences than from expensive pickup seminars.

Once you accept this reality, you turn every rejection into a win/win situation. Yes, your charms may not have won her over, but you gain valuable information and insights. Each failed approach is worth ten successful ones because true growth and learning happen outside your comfort zone.

Remember, I've been there too. When I first started putting this material into practice, I messed up countless times. Some mistakes were so significant that I crashed and burned, while others required a lot of effort to salvage the situation. Whether or not you get a number, what matters is that you're out there playing the game, living life to the fullest, and loving it.

Closing

Now let's talk about closing—what it means and how to do it correctly. Closing is more than just getting a number; it requires some technical finesse. The most crucial element is that you must do it and do it clearly and directly.

Saying something like, "Hey, nice to meet you. Maybe we should hang out sometime," is not a proper close. You need to be specific about what you want to happen next, whether it's getting her number or arranging an instant date. Surprisingly, many guys forget to close altogether. They get so pumped up about mustering the courage to approach that they rush through the interaction as quickly as possible. The conversation might go like this:

Guy: Hey, I had to stop you and tell you that you have amazing style. I love the way you put everything together.
Girl: Oh, wow, okay. Thank you.
Guy: What's your name?
Girl: Nina.
Guy: Hi, Nina. I'm George—pleased to meet you. So, what are you doing in town today?
Girl: I'm on my lunch break, actually. I'm running a bit late for work.

Guy: Okay, well, I don't want to make you late, so... um... nice to meet you.
Girl: And you.

On paper, this may sound too basic to be a common occurrence, but trust me, it happens a lot, even to me at the beginning. Let's break down this conversation and figure out why the guy failed to close the girl.

Firstly, the speed of the interaction indicates low confidence. He has self-doubt lingering in his conscious mind, which prevents him from taking the lead. The woman still holds the dominant position, and she demonstrates this by choosing to end the interaction on her terms.

She mentions being late for work, but we don't know if it's true. It could be her escape route in case this guy turns out to be a weirdo.

Even if she truly is running late, it shouldn't concern us. You should adopt the attitude that spending time with you is worth any potential earful she might receive from her boss.

If she does get in trouble at work, don't you think she'll still think it was worth it to be approached by a nice guy during her lunch break? Such encounters don't happen often for most women. Remember, you're part of an elite group since 99% of guys wouldn't have the courage to do what you're doing.

If our unlucky guy had slowed down the conversation and taken a firmer lead, he could have obtained her number before she hurried back to work.

Successful closing is all about timing. If you try to get her number before establishing rapport, she won't feel comfortable enough to share that information. This is when you're most likely to hear, "Oh, sorry, I have a boyfriend." It could mean she's genuinely unavailable, but more often, it indicates that you moved too quickly. Certain things must happen before attempting to close:

You should have talked long enough to know something about her, such as where she's from or what she's doing in town.
You should know her name, and she should know yours.
There should have been some physical contact. Likely, you shook hands when you introduced yourself, and there may have been a few light touches on the arm during the conversation.
She should have laughed or smiled at least once during the conversation. If she stood there with a stone-faced expression while you tried to work your magic, it's likely you didn't establish rapport or she's just a miserable person. In either case, you wouldn't want her number.
If you've fulfilled all these elements, you can directly ask for her number. However, the way you do it is crucial. Avoid saying something lame like, "Any chance I can get your number?" or "Would you mind if I text you later?" These statements imply that you don't expect her to comply, and you're implying that her number is of great value, which people are hesitant to give away. Instead, genuinely not caring whether she gives you her number or not, act as if you're doing her a favor by taking it.

Here are some examples:

"You seem like a cool person to hang around with. Give me your number, and I'll message you later."
"My friend is waiting for me, so I have to go, but give me your number, and we can catch up later."

"Hey, nice to meet you..." [START TO WALK AWAY, THEN DOUBLE BACK] "...I tell you what, what the hell. Give me your number, and I'll stay in touch."
There are numerous examples, but hopefully, you can see that I'm not asking for her number; I'm telling her to give it to me. If you've established yourself as the dominant member of the interaction and led the conversation, and if she has followed you this far, chances are good that she'll follow your instruction a little further.

A final word on closing: don't wait too long. Timing is everything. If you keep asking questions until you feel confident enough to ask for her number, you risk boring her or making her wonder, "What does this guy want?" Sometimes, when you wait too long, you may notice a tiny but noticeable micro-gesture of confusion flash across her face. Initially, she was fine with you approaching her, but now she's not even sure if that's what you're doing.

Repetition

"Repetition is the mother of learning, the father of action, which makes it the architect of accomplishment," as Zig Ziglar wisely said.

When you start approaching women in Day Game, the harsh reality is that, at least for a while, you're going to suck at it. There are no shortcuts to success, and personally, I'm grateful for that. If this stuff were easy, every schmuck would be doing it, and we wouldn't be in the top 1% of our gender. Game is no different from any other skill. When you learned to ride a bike, you didn't master it on the first try or even the hundredth try. As adults, we often forget how much time and effort it takes to learn something new because it's been a while since we started from scratch.

I was recently reminded of the frustrations that come with learning. A few months ago, I began studying Greek, which involved learning a new alphabet and grammar structure. My parents were planning to visit me in Cyprus in three months, and optimistically, I hoped to impress them with some basic Greek phrases. Nothing fancy, just enough to order food in restaurants and such. When I shared my ambitions with my Greek teacher, he laughed and said that maybe, with intense study for a year, I would be able to achieve that. One year! Despite having four lessons a week, the best I could hope for was basic conversation twelve months from then. I initially dismissed his comment as pessimism and dove into learning Greek, determined to prove him wrong.

Let me tell you what I've learned: Greek is ridiculously hard, especially for English speakers. You have to learn a new alphabet that is shorter than ours but has five different letters that all sound like "E." Why? There's no logical explanation. Additionally, some letters in Greek look like their counterparts in the Western alphabet but sound completely different. For example, the Greek letter "P" is pronounced as an "R." The letter "N" is spoken like an English "E." And let's not forget that Greek words have genders, but you can't guess the gender of a word. For instance, the word for "boy" in Greek is not masculine; it's neutral. All very liberal, I'm sure, but it makes the language near impossible to learn.

So, despite over twenty hours of lessons, my parents are arriving tomorrow, and I still can't speak a word of Greek. Do I believe that Greek rejected me or that Greek doesn't like me? Of course not. Greek didn't reject me; I rejected Greek. I gave up. I quit. I stopped practicing. I allowed myself to forget what I'd learned because it was too hard, too challenging, too time-consuming. I chose to focus my energy on other priorities, and that's okay. I'm not beating myself up over it. Greek wasn't essential to my life, and I have no regrets about quitting. There's no shame in quitting something that isn't bringing you joy or aligning with your goals.

Similarly, if you choose not to pursue Day Game or any other aspect of your life with women, that's entirely up to you. This book isn't intended to be a guilt trip or to make you feel inadequate. If this material doesn't resonate with you, if you don't find it enjoyable, or if you'd prefer to focus your energy elsewhere, that's fine. Life is about choices, and each choice brings us closer to or further from the life we want to live. It's entirely your decision.

With that said, if you're committed to improving your skills with women and attracting the kind of relationships you desire, repetition is key. You must be willing to put in the time and effort to practice, fail, learn, and improve. Just like riding a bike or learning Greek, it won't happen overnight, but with persistence, you'll progress. The more approaches you make, the more conversations you have, the more you put yourself out there, the more comfortable and confident you'll become.

Repetition not only allows you to refine your technique but also desensitizes you to rejection. The first few rejections might sting, but as you experience more of them, they lose their power over you. You begin to understand that rejection is not a reflection of your worth as a person but rather a result of various factors, many of which are beyond your control. With each rejection, you learn to bounce back faster, to dust yourself off, and to keep moving forward. You develop resilience and a sense of abundance, knowing that there are countless opportunities out there waiting for you.

In conclusion, detachment, closing, and repetition are essential elements in mastering Day Game. By detaching yourself from the outcome, letting go of attachment and fear of rejection, you free yourself to enjoy the present moment and embrace the valuable lessons each interaction brings. When it comes to closing, be direct and specific about what you want, ensuring that you've established rapport and timing is right. And finally, repetition is key to building your skills and desensitizing yourself to rejection, allowing you to grow and improve.

Remember, this journey is about personal growth, self-discovery, and creating meaningful connections with women. Embrace the process, learn from every experience, and most importantly, have fun along the way. Good luck!

Thank you for reading Approach And Talk To Women. If you enjoyed the book, I'd really appreciate it if you could take 30 seconds to return to the store where you purchased it and leave a rating or short review. It's one of the most powerful ways to help independent authors reach new readers.

I read every review personally, and I'm always grateful for your time and feedback.

For more in the DECODED series, along with my free True Crime Decoded podcast, visit CraigBeck.com.

Thank you for your support.

Websites:
www.CraigBeck.com
www.StopDrinkingExpert.com

Social Media
https://www.facebook.com/craigbeckbooks/
https://twitter.com/craigbeck

Other Books By Craig Beck

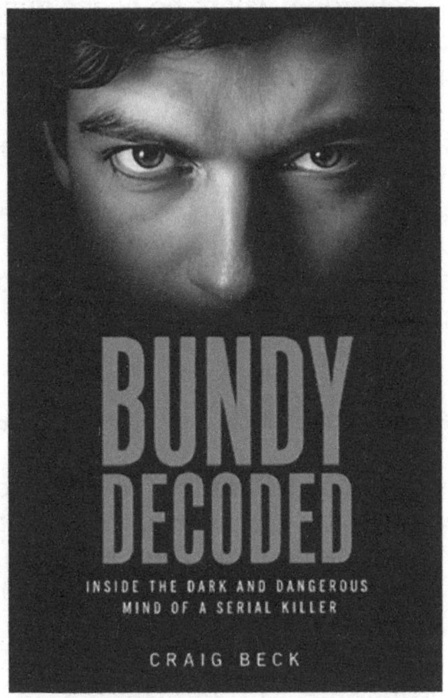

BUNDY DECODED

He was handsome, articulate, and politically ambitious. He volunteered at a suicide prevention hotline, studied law, and had a girlfriend who adored him. He also murdered at least thirty women across seven states and kept returning to their remains long after they were dead.

Ted Bundy wasn't a mystery. He was a warning.

In Bundy Decoded, bestselling author and persuasion expert Craig Beck dismantles the most famous serial killer in American history, piece by piece. This isn't another biography. This isn't a rehash of the crimes you've already read about. This is a psychological deconstruction of the man behind the mask, the childhood lie that taught him the world runs on deception, the narcissism that fuelled his double life, the escalation from voyeur to predator, and the emptiness where a conscience should have been.

From the crisis hotline where he saved lives to the sorority house where he took them. From the girlfriend who called the police and was ignored to the courtroom where he chose fame over survival. From 150 hours of death row confessions to the crowd that cheered his execution with fireworks and frying pans.

Beck goes beyond the headlines and into the wiring. How did Bundy select his victims? Why did the police have his name for years and never act? What did his own words reveal about a mind that could compartmentalise murder the way most people compartmentalise a bad day at work? And what does his story tell us about the dangerous assumptions we all carry about who we can trust?

The answer to that last question should keep you awake tonight.

Bundy Decoded is the book for readers who are done with the mythology and ready for the mechanics. It's the story of how a charming young man became a monster, told by a writer who understands that the scariest part was never the violence. It was the smile.

Available At CraigBeck.com

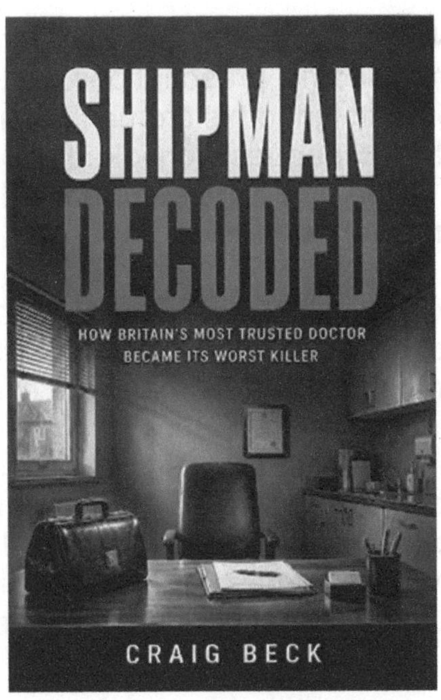

SHIPMAN DECODED

He killed more British citizens than any single criminal in history. And his patients loved him.

Harold Shipman was a family doctor in a small town in northern England. He wore glasses. He had a beard. He made house calls. He remembered your name, asked about your grandchildren, and never rushed an appointment. He was, by every measure that mattered to the people of Hyde, the best GP they'd ever had.

He was also injecting them with lethal doses of diamorphine and watching them die in their armchairs.

Two hundred and fifteen confirmed kills. Probably more. Over twenty three years, one ordinary looking man in a white coat committed the worst serial murder in modern British history, and nobody stopped him. Not the police.

Not the NHS. Not the General Medical Council. Not the pharmacists who filled his prescriptions. Not the six doctors who countersigned his cremation forms. Not the coroners. Not the colleagues who joked about his high death rate and called him "Dr Death" behind his back, then laughed it off and went home for dinner.

Shipman Decoded goes beyond the facts and into the mind. This is not a biography. This is a psychological autopsy of the most dangerous man who ever held a stethoscope, written by Craig Beck with the blunt honesty, dark humour, and razor sharp insight that his readers have come to expect. From Shipman's childhood in Nottingham and the death of his mother to the forged will that finally brought him down, this book traces the making of a killer and asks the questions that the headlines never answered.

Why did he do it? How did he choose his victims? What was happening inside his head when he sat at a dying woman's kitchen table and drank her tea? Why did every system designed to catch people like him fail so completely? And what does his story tell us about the way we trust, the way we defer, and the dangerous assumptions we make about the people who hold power over our lives?

If you think you know the Shipman story, you don't. Not until you've read this.

CraigBeck.com

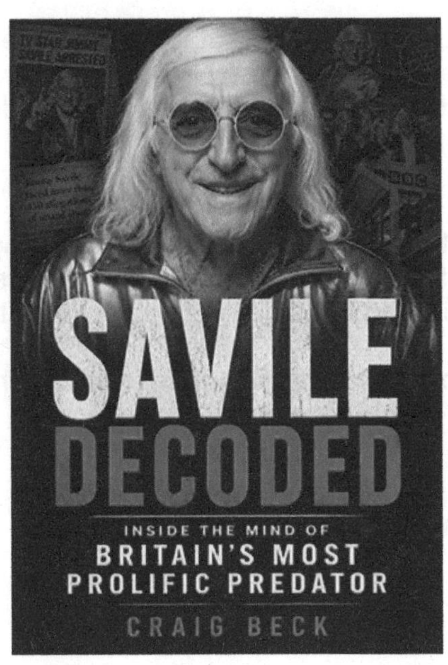

SAVILE DECODED

How did a man in a white tracksuit shake hands with the Queen on a Tuesday, visit a hospital mortuary on a Wednesday, and walk away from every investigation that ever came close to him?

For fifty years, Jimmy Savile held Britain in the palm of his hand. He raised forty million pounds for charity. He befriended a prime minister. He advised a future king. He was knighted by the Queen and honoured by the Vatican.

He was also, behind the grin and the cigar, the most prolific sexual predator in British history.

This is not a list of what he did. It is a forensic dive into why. Why he wore the costume. Why he kept five homes across five counties. Why he ran two hundred marathons. Why he volunteered, for forty years, in a hospital mortuary. Why he told a reporter, laughing, that he intended to give the country the wrong idea forever.

Every institution that should have stopped him, the BBC, the palace, the police, the church, the NHS, walked away afterwards with the same passive phrase. Mistakes were made.

By whom?

The architecture that let him operate is still standing. Somewhere tonight, a man with a laminated pass in his wallet is walking down a quiet corridor, smiling the smile the country was taught to trust.

You will never look at the safest man in the room the same way again.

CraigBeck.com

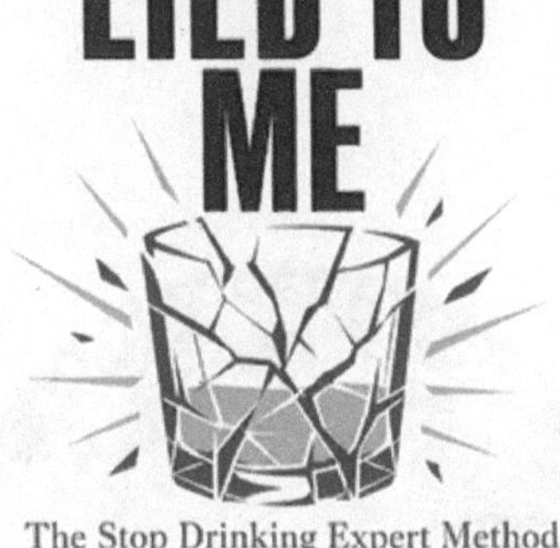

ALCOHOL LIED TO ME

My name is Craig Beck, and I am the Internet's foremost expert in helping people quit drinking alcohol. I have already helped thousands of people just like you get back in control of their drinking or stop completely. I understand how it feels to be worried about your drinking because for nearly 20 years I struggled with my own addiction. I tried everything to stop drinking alcohol from creating silly rules about what I was "allowed" to drink, and going through torturous "dry months" to taking dangerous prescription-only medication!

Absolutely nothing I tried worked until I dramatically changed my thinking. I also discovered some disturbing secrets that the alcohol industry does not want you to know. Then used my former experience as a clinical hypnotist to construct a system to help anyone get their drinking back under control. I cured my own drink problem (virtually overnight), and now I can help you stop drinking alcohol using a technique called the "Alcohol Lied to Me Method".

Available at StopDrinkingExpert.com

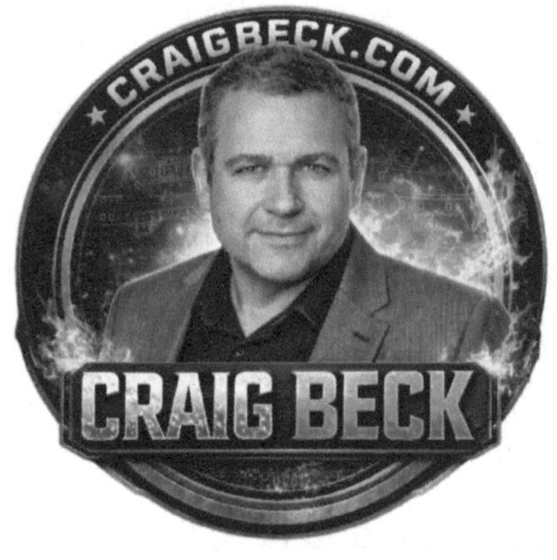

One To One Coaching With Craig Beck
Is Available At CraigBeck.com

www.ingramcontent.com/pod-product-compliance
Ingram Content Group UK Ltd.
Pitfield, Milton Keynes, MK11 3LW, UK
UKHW012255290726
14090UKWH00016B/654